Prologue

Our baby girl is starting to take her first steps. She seems a little clumsy, but that's normal for babies who are first learning how to walk. I can't believe we brought such a beautiful baby girl into this world. What a miracle! And she has an older brother that wants to protect her and take care of her. What a great world to raise two wonderful children in. I can't wait to see where their lives will take them!

6 months later…

As cute as Courtney is, she is starting to become very fussy. Now at 14 months old, she is starting to form words that are hard to understand. She is crying a lot more and starting to learn to throw temper tantrums. I can already tell the next few years will be difficult. She has been walking for a while now, but I am starting to get concerned. Although she met all the other milestones right on time, her walking doesn't seem right. She continues to walk on her toes and is falling often. I have taken her to the pediatrician, and he keeps assuring me everything is normal, and it just takes some babies extra time to grow out of their clumsiness.

3 years later

Now I am really concerned. Courtney is about to turn 4-years-old and is still walking on her tiptoes. Her preschool teachers have noticed this too and inform me that she is behind the other kids while they are running, but she manages to barely keep up with them in the running games. They assure me she fits in well with the other kids and she interacts great. She is constantly coming home with scraped up knees and elbows though. Even at home, I notice her falling, what seems like a lot, for a child her age.

I have taken her to the pediatrician and he still assures me that everything is fine. He keeps telling me that she will grow out of it and that there are no problems since she is still able to keep up with the other kids her age. As a parent, something in my gut is telling me that something's not right. I guess you can call it mother's intuition. However, the pediatrician even referred her to a pediatric neurologist in what he said would give me some peace of mind. The neurologist performed a basic exam on her and watched her walk, but she did not walk on her toes or fall in front of the neurologist. Of course, the doctors always only watch her for a few steps, so they are less likely to notice something that I, her mother, would. In fact, this time they had the nerve to suggest that I was crazy and was just trying to get attention by bringing my daughter to them. I guess it's time I stop digging in any deeper to this and wait for her to grow out of it like they say she eventually will.

Chapter 1

Imagine having a disease and not knowing about it. Growing up with something that you can't comprehend so you try to keep it hidden. Imagine one of the simplest things for you to do without thinking about and then imagine that simple thing taking every ounce of strength that you can conquer up just to complete a simple task.

All my life I've grown up with some type of problem not knowing what it was. For as long as I can remember I've struggled with weak muscles in my legs while the rest of me was "normal." The problem is mostly with my legs and quadriceps muscles. For example, a "normal" person can kneel or squat on the ground and get up no problem without even thinking about the motions they are enacting. Then there's me; I can't. For me to get up I must use the muscle strength in my arms to push up to a standing position. From the time I was old enough to be in school, maybe even before, this has always been my biggest insecurity and the one thing I am most self-conscious about. I would often find myself wondering what is wrong with me and if I can ever fix it. My entire life mission has been based around trying to gain strength and working towards a goal of standing up from the floor without using my arms and running an entire mile without stopping.

When it comes to school, it has always been easy for me, except when it came to P.E. Unfortunately, problems with muscles is something you can't hide, no matter how hard you try. The other kids would laugh and tease me about the way I would run or how I couldn't keep up with them. My endurance has always been lacking and anytime there was some sort of physical competition, I would always come in last place. Nobody wanted me on their team during class. They would mock the way I ran and tease me about gasping for air as I would try to catch my breath. They would push me over or trip me whenever they had a chance. I guess they feared I would drag them down too, which now I can understand, but at the time it really hurt my feelings. I spent many nights crying myself to sleep and every day I would come home and wonder, "Why me? Why did God have to make me this way?" Then I would think, "If I could just be "normal" everything will be okay." I didn't let their torture stop me though, I still did everything any other "normal" kid would do.

Ironically, I loved playing sports, except I hated running. I started out doing gymnastics. I loved doing summersaults and cartwheels and the flips always amazed me. I would have butterflies in my stomach before every performance and I'd imagine myself in front of an audience every time I stepped onto the balance beam. Soon after, I started doing martial arts. This turned out to be the best thing that could have happened in my life. I was 5-years-old and my big brother was doing it, so naturally I wanted to also. I don't remember the exact details for why I started, but that's the one thing I fell in love with through the entirety of my childhood. I spent 15 years practicing Tae Kwon Do. All those years with the kids mocking me, I would transform my anger and my feelings into each technique. Thinking back on it now, I'm still amazed that I was able to be as successful as I was in the art without knowing what was up.

Aside from martial arts, I played soccer for six years, softball for two, and basketball for another two years. Basketball was my favorite of those, but once I got to junior high, I didn't want to try out for the team. I was most afraid of the stories I heard about practice and all the running involved. I was scared I wouldn't be able to endure it and keep up with my classes. I also didn't want to quit martial arts, so I joined the marching band instead. There I found I wasn't so coordinated with marching while playing a musical instrument. When the instructor kept asking me if I could hear the beat of the drums and repeating over and over that I needed to keep my march to the beat of the drum I wanted to cry. I was giving 100% effort and no matter how much I tried I could not stay in form with the rest of the band. This is when I knew I needed to give up being in a marching band.

Starting junior high school, my condition really became a problem. Now I had a full class period dedicated to exercise. We had to run, almost every single day, and I always had people asking me if I was hurt, including the teachers. People have described it to me as my legs looking stiff and that it looks like I'm limping while I'm running. Not only that, but I am also lacking in endurance, so I was always finish last. It didn't make it easy to fit in with your classmates when everyone asked if something was wrong with you and you didn't have a clue what to say. I remember when we all had to take the mile test and every single person that had P.E. the same period lapped me. I remember running my last lap completely solo and all the P.E. teachers got their classes to cheer me on while I was running. Although this was a motivation tactic, for me I was humiliated. Everyone was staring at me while I ran and based on previous experiences a felt like half the seventh grade was mocking me. After that class, I went to the bathroom to hide while I cried about that experience. Something else that happened that year during physical education was everyone had to partner up and sit back to back with their partner, with linked arms. Then we had to collaborate with our partner to stand up at the same time. Well, as you can probably guess, that didn't go very well. Not only could I not stand up, but I was holding my partner back as well so he couldn't stand either and he yelled at me about not standing up. I left class crying that day too because of course, my partner was the guy I liked at that time. In a 13-year-old girl's mind, the world came crashing down that day. Now I never had a chance for him liking me back and I didn't think I would ever have a boyfriend because rumors spread fast and everyone would know my secret. Even though I was considered smart in all my classes, I still had people that treated me like I was stupid in all my classes. They told me that I would never be good at anything since I couldn't perform at a "normal" athletic level. Next came high school, where things became even more intense.

The first day of my freshman year my P.E. class is where I really noticed I wouldn't be able to keep my secret hidden as much as I wanted to. The first day that we ran in class my teacher stopped me after one lap because he wanted to talk to me. He asked what was wrong with me and why I was running the way I was and if I was okay. I told him that I was okay and as far as I know there was nothing wrong with me. In reality, I was okay, but I probably could have given more details and explained my situation. I think if I had he probably would have been able to help me out, had I not been trying to hide that part of myself. Honestly, that is one of my biggest regrets; not being more honest about my capabilities, or in this case incapability's. I never was able to run a full mile, but that P.E. teacher helped me out a lot. When star testing rolled around, instead of having me run the mile test, he kept working with me to run the pacer test. I forget how many times I had to take it until I passed, but I do remember I was at a point where I was about to give up and give into failing P.E. He started running with me encouraging me to keep going and to keep up with his pace. Looking back on it now, that is one of the nicest, most helpful things that any of my teachers have ever done to help me.

Sophomore year rolled around and facing my P.E. class every day became even more of a challenge. My teacher that year was the coach of the football team and most of my classmates were star athletes. I don't remember anyone ever saying anything to me that year, but I always felt like my class was judging me. They probably thought I was just being lazy. I would start off jogging every time we had to run and about halfway through, my jog would fade into a walk. Whenever we would play sports in class, I was always the last one picked for the team because no one wanted someone as clumsy as me on their team. One day we were playing volleyball and I hit the ball in a completely different direction than I wanted it to go in. The ball hit the teacher in the back of the head and the teacher told the class that the next person to hit him with the ball would get detention. Well guess what, I hit him in the head a second time while he had his back turned. I'm sure my face was bright red as I was dying from embarrassment and my partner that day was in hysterics. The teacher kept asking who did it and luckily, everyone in the class stayed silent. I was that clumsy and I think one of the worst things would have been getting a detention due to my clumsiness.

I can understand that with a competitive class no one would want me on their team, but it still came with an impact on my self-esteem. I didn't want to participate, but I knew I had to, and doing so led me into a deep depression.

My biggest relief came junior year when I was no longer forced to take a P.E. class. However, by that time, I had also stopped taking martial arts classes. I planned to find a job so I could pay for the classes myself after getting my driver's license. This is exactly what I did and a good motivator for me to find my first job. I started working at the local box chain retailer as a cashier. As my homework piled up a little more every day, my work hours began to expand, and by the end of the week, I was exhausted. Eventually, I would notice sometimes after sitting for a long period of time, then standing up, my legs would just give out on me and I would fall to the ground. It was almost like my legs turned into jelly and I would crash down or reach for something to hold onto before they would reappear as my legs. I thought about getting checked out, but every time I thought about it, I stopped myself and told myself it would only hurt my parents to know I was curious.

By the middle of my junior year I was working 25 hours per week, taking martial arts classes, taking a class at the junior college, a member of a school club, driving everywhere I went, and going on dates with my boyfriend on the weekends. All are completely normal activities for an average sixteen-year-old. However, it was exhausting and overwhelming for me. After every Tae Kwon Do class, I would be so sore the next day that I wasn't sure if I would be able to move. Even though I lived within walking distance of my high school, I made the choice to start driving. This was mostly because of the guys that would always walk behind me and mock the way I walked. I always thought it was fun to wave at them walking to school while I was driving my car. Gradually, I started noticing things that made me think any muscle strength I had was growing weaker.

In the middle of my senior year, after I was accustomed to driving everywhere, I could tell my muscles were growing weaker and weaker. Walking across campus was becoming a struggle for me. I would start feeling tired by the time I reached my next class. Luckily, class periods gave me a break and a reason to sit down. Then one day in my anatomy and physiology class my teacher decided to have us do an experiment testing each other's reflexes. I was extremely lucky that one of my best friend's was in class with me and completely understanding of my situation. Also, she was my partner for this experiment. When it came time to test the leg reflexes by banging the knee with a hammer, neither of my legs budged so my friend thought she was doing something wrong. We called the teacher over and she tried herself. It appeared I did have the reflex, but it was extremely weak. This is when I first began to wonder how much longer I could keep my secret hidden from the rest of the world.

Not only did I feel like I was going through this completely alone, but I also felt like nobody would ever understand, no matter how hard I tried explaining it to them. My friends tried as hard as they could to understand, but really, how could they when they didn't know what it was like to not have muscles. I felt more alone than ever. My family, especially my brother (an athlete) kept telling me how lazy I was becoming. Every movement felt like it was becoming

more of a struggle each day. My boyfriend at the time
didn't help either by telling me that I was very lazy and that
I didn't try hard enough. We had several other
disagreements as well and our age difference at the time
didn't help. He was a freshman in college struggling to
keep up with his classes and life pressures, while I was
trying to find the energy to have fun and enjoy my senior
year. This meant that I had a lot of free time on my hands
while he was always busy. He rarely returned my calls and
when we did hang out, he would call me names for not
giving in to having sex with him, even though he knew
where I stood on the matter before we had started dating.
This was tearing me down and making me feel bad about
myself. For this reason, among others, I decided it would
be best to end things between us. Even though I had broken
up with him, he was my very first love and I was
devastated. I battled with depression and constantly thought
about ending my life. I didn't see the point of living and I
didn't think I would ever be able to fall in love again. I was
wrong.

During the summer after my senior year, I spent the days
becoming close friends with one of my coworkers. He was
always making me laugh and really caring, sweet, and
sensitive. He was also outgoing, something I'm not, and I
really liked how he wasn't scared to be himself. Once I
started my first semester of college in the fall, he had
become my best friend. I felt I could tell him anything. I
told him my biggest, darkest secrets and he told me his. It
turned out that as much as we were different, we also had a
lot in common. I'm not sure how or why, but I was easily
able to open up to him. I told him about my muscle
weakness and how I didn't know what it was and how I had
constantly thought about ending my life and all my

sleepless nights. He assured me that I am a great person, and no one could take that away from me. He also supported me while I worked out and encouraged me to do my best. He hugged me tight and made me promise him that anytime I started to feel like that I would call him. He showed me that I did have a purpose and a reason to live. For that, I still feel like I owe him my life.

As our lives grew even busier and our friendship stronger, my feelings for him were starting to show even more. I wasn't sure if I should tell him or not. I had so many reasons not to, but love took over my heart and one day I showed him a poem I had written about my feelings for him. To my relief, he felt the same way and we no longer had to keep our love for each other a secret. The more we spent time together, the more our love grew deeper and stronger for one another. We did everything together and I told him everything. He was very understanding and very helpful. Anytime I started getting tired he understood and would let me take it easy and try to help me in any way he could. I felt this was one of the sweetest things that anyone had ever done for me, but it also meant my muscles were getting used to taking it easy and were deteriorating a little bit more.

Eventually the unimaginable happened and we started growing apart. I saw a different side of him, and I didn't want to tell him what was wrong because I was afraid of hurting his feelings. I just stopped talking to him like I used to. I stopped letting him in and started to push him away. He sensed that something was off, but neither of us wanted to talk about it. The night he broke up with me was one of the hardest experiences so far in my life. Sitting in the parking lot he told me that he loved me and that I was his best friend. He told me that I am beautiful, inside and out, and not to ever let anyone tell me differently. Then it came out. We talked about us and agreed it was time to end our relationship. Then he made me promise that no matter what happened between us that we would always be friends and that I would never take my own life. Even though we no longer keep in touch, that is the one promise to him I keep.

After our break up, we had agreed to remain as friends, but when he contacted me the next day asking if I could have lunch with him, I turned him down. I couldn't stop crying that week and I didn't want him to see me that way. About a week later, a few people had confirmed what I had tried to erase from my mind several weeks prior. He had been cheating on me and that's when again I felt my whole world was crashing down. I had thought we might be able to get through this time and still be close friends. After all, not long ago we were talking about planning a wedding. My heartfelt like it had been ripped to pieces, torn out of my chest, stitched back together, just to be broken again. At that moment I knew our friendship would never be the same because I would never be able to trust him.

After that time period, I fell into the deepest depression that I had experienced at that point in my life. I did become very lazy and never wanted to go out or do anything. I should also add I hated my job, as an assistant manager at a horrible shoe store, during this time period which did not help with my emotions. Then the days that I would go out, I would immediately start crying because everything reminded me of him, and our time spent together. He was the person I needed the most during that time, but I knew seeing him would only make matters worse. There were so many times I felt like just giving up and somedays I would even take a bottle of pills with me to my room. One night I even got as far as emptying the bottle into my hand and taking a couple. As I was swallowing them, I thought of the promise I made to him, then of the way he broke his promise to me. Then I thought about my grandma and how she would say she was so disappointed in me if I met her in Heaven. Then I thought of the alternative. And finally, I thought about how my parents would find me and all the secrets I had been keeping. After the 3 pills I had taken, I poured the rest back into the bottle. That night, I decided I had reason to keep living. Even though I never told my family my thoughts or actions, I was very lucky to have their love and support and that of my friends as well to help me surpass those hard times. Now, my ex and I are connected through social media, and from time to time I have thought about messaging him, but while "she" is still in his life that is a road I'm not willing to go down.

Although it's been tough, these experiences have led me to where I am today. I feel like I have really grown up and become a different person from the person I once was. Now, I'm considering dating again, but first I want to focus on completely improving myself and discover who I am. These are the reasons I am here. I am finally ready to look for answers and release my secret into the world.

Chapter 2 (3 years later)

New Year's Eve has rolled around once again. In my life, I have never been more nervous and anxious as I am right now. This is the year I am deciding to finally take care of myself and find an understanding for who I am. 2014 is going to be a challenging year, but in the end it will be worth it. My work hours have finally returned to early morning shifts instead of all-nighters. I can't remember the last time I had this much energy. It feels as if everything is starting to fall into place and for once in my life, everything feels like things are going right.

Leaving work at a quarter to nine, the morning sunbeams against my face and the warmth helps set a happy tone. My manager had asked me to stay, and of course I feel a little guilty saying no as there was plenty work to be done, but I did inform him that I have a doctor's appointment. His caring nature asked if everything was okay and if I was just going in for a checkup, which I said I was as I wasn't ready to dive into my entire life story. As I'm walking out the sliding doors, the morning breeze chills my skin as I'm walking towards my aged Pontiac. I'm grinning from ear to ear because today is the first day I'm taking a step to discover a part of me that has always been present, but never identified. This is a part of me I have kept secret so long, and today, I am deciding to put it out in the open, so I no longer have to wonder what's going on with me.

Next thing I know, a woman's voice calls my name, "Courtney, come on back." I follow the nurse back to the room smelling of blood and filled with medical supplies. She wraps the blue cuff around my arm, and it squeezes until a quiet beep is heard. Simultaneously, a short metal stick is placed under my tongue where a louder beep is shortly heard after the faint sound from the blood pressure machine. The nurse assures me my vitals are normal then asks the dreaded question, "What brings you in today, Courtney?"

"I have been having problems with balance," I simply state. At this moment I realize I have just given a front-row seat to a talent I've tried to keep hidden for so long. The nurse excuses herself and assures me that Hannah will be in shortly.

Sure enough, almost as soon as the nurse leaves, I hear a hollow knocking on the exam door before it swings open. An older woman with shoulder-length, silver hair enters, "Hello, I'm Hannah; a physician's assistant here at Ellie Clinic. You must be Courtney."

"Hi Hannah, it's nice to meet you," I quiver shaking her hand gazing directly into her deep brown eyes.

"What seems to be the problem?"

"Balance," I retort as I go on to tell her my background information. I inform her of how I notice that I am constantly tripping over my own two feet and how I am often falling over and getting knocked off my feet. I mention that some of my friends, as well as strangers, have commented on how sometimes I seem to be limping as I walk. Although, I leave out the time a stranger gave me directions to an emergency room because of the way I was walking.

She asks if I have any pain or dizziness, in which I continue to tell her about my past experiences with sports and how I think my balance issues are a result of muscle weakness. I inform Hannah that even though I have dealt with these issues all my life, I would really like to find out what has been causing it. I explain that I have been thinking about my future and have been wondering about having children of my own someday and if they could be affected. After taking a detailed medical history of any former injuries and of any known diseases that run in my family, the professional has me hop onto the exam table so she can perform some tests.

First things first, Hannah looks at the bottom of my shoes and explains that by looking at them, she can see how they are worn out a little differently on each side, showing that my gait is abnormal. Next, she has me remove my shoes and socks before asking me to lay back on the cold, narrow table. This is where she takes my right leg and places it in a parallel position to the floor. From here, she places her hand on my foot and tells me that while she is pushing into work against her, so she won't be able to push my leg in. My leg is able to resist and strengthens against the pressure of her cold hands. Then the same thing is done with my left leg with the same results. After a short, awkward silence, Hannah has me sit up and tells me now she will do the same thing, and wants me to push against her like before, but in a different area. This time she rests her hands against my leg, in the spot under where my knee is bent and tells me to kick out, not letting her push my leg back in. Barely able to swing my leg out without any resistance, this comes as a great struggle for me. However, I am able to resist Hannah's pressure on my left leg for a short amount of time. With my right leg, I couldn't swing my leg out at all. Next, the physician assistant has me attempt to lift each leg into the air, neither one lifting more than a couple centimeters. Finally, Hannah has me perform one last difficult test while I am sitting on the exam table. She tells me to watch her as she takes one leg, picks it up and touches her knee to her ankle, before sliding it in a controlled motion down her shin. "Now, I would like for you to do the same thing with one leg and then the other," she instructed. Just lifting my ankle to my opposite knee is an extremely difficult task and I'm barely able to touch my left leg at all while sliding my right leg down in a very jerky movement. Repeating this motion with my left leg is still a challenge, but the motion is a little more controlled.

Once these torturous strength tests come to an end, Hannah informs me that it is time to check my reflexes. First, she takes her anvil and slides it across the bottom of my feet. Next, she bangs a medical hammer against my kneecap, testing my patellar reflex on both sides, but neither returns a result. This time she tells me to clasp my hands together and when she says go to try pulling them apart, but without letting them come detached from each other. She has me close my eyes while doing this and she tries the patellar reflex test again. Still, no results were yielded from this experiment. Hannah lets out a quiet sigh and tells me to stand up. At this point, I don't know what to think, but for the first time in my life I am seeing a look of wonder and a look of disappointment that I have never seen from a medical professional. Not sure what to do, I study her body language and facial expressions trying to grasp any clues of what might be going through her mind as I continue to follow her directions.

The physician assistant watches closely as I place each hand beside me on the table and use the muscles in my arms to push my body into a standing position. Hannah then asks me to walk across the room on my toes, turn around, and walk back the same way. This was easy for me and I didn't notice anything out of the ordinary, after all, I do remember my mom saying that I used to always walk on my toes as a young child. The hard part comes next as she tells me to do the same thing, except this time walk on my heels. I start to lean back onto my heels, but as soon as I rock back and try to release the weight from the balls of my feet, I lose my balance and start to fall over. Luckily, she catches me before my knees start to tremble and I am able to regain my balance.

She tells me to continue anyway, so I rock back to my heels not releasing all the weight from the balls of my feet and rock back and forth as much as I can without hitting the ground. After this agony concludes, Hannah has me follow her out of the exam room and into the hallway. Here, she watches me walk my normal every day walk back and forth down the long hallway. It may be a little different from my normal walk because I am feeling self-conscious about how I was walking this time, with other people occasionally passing through. Sometimes when I know someone is watching the way I walk, I subconsciously try to walk what my brain has deemed as a normal walk. Hannah stands in complete silence after this walking fiasco and leads me back into the small room. I am instructed to sit back on the table, so I lift myself using my arms once again. From here, she hands me my tennis shoes and socks and tells me to put them on. As I do this she stares through her metal-rimmed glasses watching every detail; the way my hands are shaking a little, how I lift my left leg and cross it over my right to put my garments on that foot, how I lift my right leg with the help of my hand, and the way I tie my shoes, making one loop, then going around and pulling the string back through the loop. Next, she tells me to step off the table and have a seat in the chair next to the desk within the room.

Once I'm seated, Hannah goes on to explain my options, "You can do one of two things; go see a physical therapist or go to a neurologist."

At this point, I realize I just invited an audience into a viewing of my darkest secret. "Can a physical therapist determine what is causing this," I inquire and explain I would like to have children one day, but I don't want to pass anything on to them. She informs me that a physical therapist would be able to work with me to increase my strength, but only a neurologist could find the cause. Then Hannah tells me that due to my age and the way my shoes are worn it's possible I might have an early onset of Multiple Sclerosis (M.S.) or Amyotrophic Lateral Sclerosis (ALS). Once I hear those words, my heart sinks. I know that neither has a cure and either one would mean that I won't have any hope in gaining strength within my legs. She does tell me that she's not saying I do, but a neurologist would be able to do the testing and determine what is going on, while a physical therapist would only be able to help to increase my strength. I agree to see a neurologist because at this point, I want answers. I also have been exercising on my own, and not gaining strength with my exercises when I know any other person doing the same routine would have gained strength.

Since my health care plan is a PPO and I want to see someone in the same county as me rather than driving further, she suggests I see Dr. Bronco and writes down his phone number for me to set up an appointment. At this point, Hannah hands me her card and asks me to give it to the neurologist so they can let her know what is going on with me. She also asks me to send her an e-mail and keep her updated with my condition and any progress with the neurologist as she is curious about what it might be. I thank her and say I will keep her updated before saying goodbye before returning to my car. The thirty-second elevator ride to the downstairs portion of the office building feels like a lifetime as I'm pushing back tears, trying to not show emotion with the other elevator rider that only wanted to make small conversation. The elevator doors swing open and I hurry out, almost running, to the outside of the building. My car is within a few steps from the office entryway and as I open my car door tears immediately roll down my face. I sit in my car, staring out the windshield, tears streaming down my face, for a good half hour before I start my engine. My life as I have always known it is coming to an end and I don't know what I am thinking or feeling in this very moment.

Chapter 3

With the news I just received, I felt things were tumbling in. Nothing would ever be the same again. As I was driving home rivers of tears continued to stream down my face. I could barely see where I was going or what was in front of me, but I didn't care. I thought about crashing my car into the trees and praying for the end, then I thought about the possibility of harming someone else. I didn't want an innocent bystander to be placed in harm's way because of the way I was feeling. I also thought about what a waste that would be to my beautiful, sporty car and how I had promised to drive all my friends to a party tonight. My brain was all over the place, jumping from thought to thought. I pulled in front of my house in a calm manner, trying to take deep breaths. Once I reached the door of my house, I tried my best to force the tears back in. I didn't want anyone to know or see the condition I was in. I didn't want anyone to ask questions or know what they had said at my doctor's appointment until I knew for sure what was going on. I wipe the tears from my eyes, take a long, slow deep breath and push the door open.

Walking through the house, purse in hand, I head straight to the computer room. Here, I close the door and look closely at the small piece of paper Hannah had given me with the name of a neurologist, Dr. George Bronco, (545) 555-4782. I stare at this for a long minute before reaching for my cell phone to dial the number. Unfortunately, an automated service answers and informs me that this number is no longer in service, then suggests other numbers for different people I might be trying to reach, but Dr. Bronco's name is never mentioned. So, I do what anyone would do, head into the computer room, boot up the old machine, and go straight to google where I type in his name. Only the same number continues to pop up, so at this point, I'm not sure what to do. I call my general physician's office back and alert them to the neurologist situation. They inform me that because my plan is a PPO I can call my insurance company and ask for the name of a neurologist that would be covered in my plan and to call them again and let them know what I find.

Instead of calling, I decided to check online. Once I reach my healthcare plan's website, I search through a list of neurologists when finally, one person with a special interest in balance problems catches my eye. I click on Dr. Bobby Manteca's name which takes me to his profile. As I'm reading through the information, I discover he has a special interest in Multiple Sclerosis, balance disorders, and muscle disorders. I'm already convinced this neurologist is for me, but as I continue scanning through the page, I see he is also a martial artist. Now I know, he is perfect for my needs. So, I give his office a call and try to set up an appointment, but the receptionist tells me I can't schedule an appointment without a referral. Here, I do the logical thing and call Hannah's office back. I leave a message on their answering machine that I found a neurologist I would like to see, but Dr. Manteca won't accept patients without a referral. I give them all the information and decide to follow up after the new year. I specifically ask them to call back on my cell phone number to maintain my privacy, instead of the household number they have had on file since before I was of legal age. This may also be why I waited so long to request assistance in figuring out what was wrong with me; before I turned 18 and I had an appointment at that office, they called my mom to ask for permission to treat me when I was 16. Talk about scaring a teenager away from any necessary medical treatments or options.

Becoming more nervous from receiving the news I had been given this morning, I decide I will tell all my closest friends since we are all going to a party later, instead of keeping it locked inside like I had originally planned. However, within a few minutes, my mom is asking me why I was referred to see a neurologist and what is going on. I am completely in shock at this point and demand to know how she knows. She plays the message on the household answering machine that Hannah's office had left for me. It was from the receptionist calling to say they had received my message and will send a referral right over. They had completely ignored my request to only call on my cell phone number. At this point, I have to open up and tell my mom that I finally decided to ask why I wasn't getting stronger. My entire life, she had made me feel like I needed to hide that part of myself by not talking to me about it, and now here it is all out in the open. While I was irate with the office, I didn't know what to do, and was in a foul mood before the party. I couldn't wait to get out of my house, like anyone in my position would want an escape.

 Once Jessie arrives, I drive her and Kallie to Daisy's house. We were the first people to arrive which gave me the perfect opportunity to share my news. "Guys, I have something to tell you," I say with a shaky voice. As soon as I have their attention, I continue, "So I went to my doctor this morning because I am finally going to find out what is wrong with me after all these years. As it turns out, I have to see a neurologist because my doctor things I possibly have M.S. or ALS."

Honestly, this isn't very clear to me, so I don't remember exactly what I said, but I do remember everyone being supportive and understanding. Shortly after I tell everyone, we decide everyone else was taking too long to arrive, so we might as well start eating. By the time I finally finished eating I had 10 slices of pizza (an entire pizza). My friends were all laughing at how skinny I am and how I ate the most. Then we decide that it's New Year's Eve, we had a ton of alcohol, so why not just get started drinking. Just wanting to forget everything about this day and start over, I thought this was a great idea.

I start slow with some Vodka mixed with a green jolly rancher soda. All of us sit around talking and watching TV while slowly sipping our drinks. Once these are finished, we go back for more. This time, I still have Vodka, but I mixed it with watermelon flavored soda, about half and half. Soon more people started showing up, nobody that I knew, so the shy side of me took over and I just stand quietly drinking in the background. Starting to feel a little dizzy halfway through this drink I sit down in an empty chair next to Jessie. Not long after, I hear Kallie say, "Come on Courtney, you're being too quiet."

"Ya, I know," I reply somewhat annoyed. Not wanting to come off as a complete quiet stranger to everyone, I think drinking a little more might help to release the out-going version of me so I down the rest of my drink. Before I know what's going on, Jessie is pouring the rest of her drink into my cup because she doesn't like it, so I down that too. Next thing I know, someone hands me a whiskey shot, which I take like a champ, all in one gulp. This is my first party and I don't know what the norm is, so I don't want to look completely out of place, when I am already feeling completely uncomfortable in this atmosphere. On top of everything else, I am also trying to hide the news I received this morning, because this was the biggest insecurity from my lifetime, and I don't want anyone I don't know to know what I'm experiencing.

Pretty soon everyone is heading into the living room to play beer pong, so I stand up to go in and watch. At this point, I'm still feeling dizzy, but it's not any worse than earlier, so of course I wanted to play too. First, I cheer on Jessie as she plays and try to figure out the rules. Next thing I know, I'm up and my partner is a guy named Cliff. Mind you, before tonight I had only played once in my life and I had sucked at it then. It was also in a different atmosphere, with Jessie as my partner and with lots of rules. In the beginning, I am horrible and need to keep drinking the beer. As the game continues, the better I get, and I am starting to become extremely drunk from all of the previous drinks beforehand. By the time we were finished, I had drunk four cups of beer and I don't remember which team won. All I know is the room was starting to spin so I needed to find somewhere to sit down. The empty seat on the couch next to me made the perfect spot, so I sat down watching and cheering while this time Jessie played.

After beer pong ceased, it was time to go into the kitchen for some tequila shots. If anyone informed me that we were waiting for everyone to get a shot in their hands, I never heard them. As soon as Daisy handed me the shot, I drank it, then everyone asked why I didn't wait. I shrugged it off explaining I didn't realize what we were doing and asked for another. This time, I waited to drink it. As I took a step back, I nearly fell over, so I sit down at the table not realizing they were about to play another drinking game.

Thinking everyone at the table had to play when Cliff asked if I was going to play, I said yes. If felt weird being the only girl playing, but all the guys were really sweet and kept explaining the rules as we played. By this time, I'm pretty sure Daisy and Jessie were watching me intensely. It turned out, I was really good at this game though and only had to drink one cup of beer.

As soon as this game is over, I step back and would have fallen over if Daisy didn't catch me. Falling all over myself, in a different manner than normal, made Jessie ask if I felt like I was going to throw up or if I was okay. At first, I felt fine, but then it hit me. Cliff and Ben helped me into the bathroom since all my friends were too short to match my height. They were about to drop me on the floor when Jessie explained to set me down gently because I have a muscle disorder and she didn't think I'd be able to catch myself. Next thing I know, someone is tying back my hair. Jessie stayed with me however long I was in that position, until someone said they needed in the bathroom. At this point, Jessie went to find Ben so he and Daisy could help me up. The two of them barely helped me to the doorstep before I collapsed laughing. I think it's safe to say that night, I may have forgotten what I was trying to forget.

The fresh air felt great with a gentle breeze blowing cold air against my face, but I started worrying about what the neighbors might think. Jessie came outside with water and helped me sit up and stay out of the bushes that I kept trying to roll in. At this point, Jessie started feeding me bread and making me drink water. The reaction made me feel sick. Finally, the restroom was free again and Cliff was standing in front of me. Since I was sitting on a step, all I remember is wrapping my arms around his neck and I remember saying that I was giving him a hug. He told me to keep hugging him and once I was completely leaning against him as he used his strength to stand up and pull me to my feet. By this time, I think he was a bit drunk too, and when we reached the small square room, all I remember are my knees banging against the hard, cold tile. Next thing I know, Jessie is telling me that it's midnight, I made it to the new year. I quietly said, "Happy New Year" and all I remember is waking up on the couch the next morning.

When I awake, my straight hair is turned into a puffball, completely made of static and I feel like crap! I open my eyes and the room is spinning in circles and I become extremely nauseous. When I try to sit up, I am immediately running to the bathroom. Pretty soon, everyone else awakes and starts talking about going to Denny's to get food. Normally Denny's serves as a great hangover food for me, but this time the thought of being in a moving vehicle made me rush into the restroom again. Although eating something sounded like a good idea to me, I decided to stay behind. Although, I did ask them to bring me back a banana and some Gatorade.

While everyone else was out, I took the opportunity to go back to sleep. Even though it took everyone about two hours to return it felt like five minutes. They gave me a Gatorade and a bag of chips. I took a sip of the sports drink, then began digging into the chips. About halfway through the bag, I find my way back to the bathroom floor. Once I start feeling better, we decide it is time to head home before another wave of nausea strikes. Since I was am still dizzy and my head is still pounding, we decide it will be best for Jessie to drive my car home.

When we walk inside, my mom shakes her head, and my dad laughs at Kallie and I. Still hungry, I start eating a banana. After that went down fine, I decide to eat a real meal. Still feeling horrible, I wasn't sure what would be a good idea to try, so I make a smoothie with my Gatorade to help replenish my electrolytes. Then I decide to sleep for the rest of the day and hopefully the hangover will eventually disappear.

In the coming weeks, things are starting to get shaky and flashbacks start playing like a movie in my mind. Over and over again, the moment Hannah mentioned MS or ALS rolled through my brain like a never-ending story. Then memories of everything from that night and day keep popping up, like the flashbacks in a movie. Memories I had no recollection of came into my mind. It kind of feels like I'm the star of my own movie, with some parts removed and a different actress replacing me.

Chapter 4

After what feels like an eternity, the day of my neurology appointment finally arrives. I am nervous as can be, but ecstatic that for the first time in my entire life I will possibly receive some insight into what is wrong with me, finally. Jessie previously mentioned she would be willing to come with me to help explain some things about the way I walk and things I have told her about my muscle situation. Since I can extremely forgetful and not always the best at explaining things and I can't see the way I walk, I graciously accepted her presence. Since my appointment is at 9 am and I am not sure how long it will take to drive in the morning traffic and find the facility, I leave my house and pick Jessie up around 8 am. There isn't a lot of traffic, so we end up finding the medical building around 8:30 am. Still having thirty minutes to spare, we decide to quickly grab a bite to eat at the nearby McDonald's since both of us are starving by this point, as neither of us had a chance to eat before leaving our houses.

As we walk into the gigantic medical facility I am immediately overwhelmed. Stairs can be seen upon entering, as well as several office buildings and long always. I guess I must look lost as well because pretty soon I hear a voice saying, "What are you looking for?" as I'm trying to navigate all of the directional signs.

"Where is neurology?" I asked with a shaky voice, still nervous about someone that I might know seeing me and overhearing my conversation with the kind assistant.

"Upstairs," they replied, "Take the elevators in the back behind the stairs and the neurology department will be on your left." I thank them and Jessie and I walk into the elevators and ride up. My knees are shaking so much, and I have to hold onto the bar against the elevator wall to keep my balance. My heart is racing and while part of me is ready for this appointment to take place, the other part of me is scared to death and wants to run away from this very moment. Once the elevator doors open and we step out, the big sign for neurology and the check-in desk is immediately to our left, just as the kind gentleman downstairs had told us. I walk up to the desk, "Hello, my name is Courtney Cowmen. I have an appointment with Dr. Manteca at 9 am," still shaking and not ready for this moment.

"Hi Courtney. It's nice to meet you. I just have some forms for you to fill out before being seen," as he hands me a paper to sign about the HIPPA Privacy Act. I then sign a couple of other forms and the kind receptionist informs me because I was am still early to have a seat in the waiting area and they will call me back shortly. At this, I go and take a seat next to Jessie, still filling out the first-time patient form, checking the box for muscle weakness and asking Jessie to help me describe anything that needs a description. While we are waiting, I notice the initials D.O. next to Dr. Manteca's name instead of the usual M.D. Curiosity gets the best of me, so Jessie helps me to look up what the letters mean since my hands are too shaky to function for anything else. We learn that the D.O. holds an osteopathic medical degree which means the doctor takes more of a holistic approach to medicine and is concerned with treating the whole patient instead of only the patient's symptoms. After a short time, the nurse calls me in, so I introduce Jessie and asked if she can come back with me, explaining that she is my best friend and she is here for support. He agrees and introduces himself as Avery, before leading us into a large room with a chair, instead of the typical patient table seen in generic medical offices. After I get settled in he takes my vitals and lets me in, "Everything looks good," before asking, "What brings you in today?" I quickly summarize my muscle weakness and balance issues in the fewest sentences as possible, and he informs me the doctor will be in shortly.

Soon we hear a shallow knock at the door. A tall, middle-aged gentleman steps inside, "Hello, I am Dr. Manteca."

"Nice to meet you, I'm Courtney, and this is my friend Jessie," I greet back.

"Nice to meet you," he shakes both of our hands before he turns to me and asks, "What brings you in today?"

"I have been having lots of problems with balancing and tripping over things and I fall a lot. I think it's because my leg muscles are extremely weak and I would like to find out why, when I am constantly working out trying to get them stronger. I would also like to know if I will be able to have kids of my own one day and if they will be affected."

"Does anyone in your family have a history of neurological disorders? Or has anyone in your family experienced any signs of muscle weakness that you know of?"

"Only Alzheimer's."

"Hmm, that doesn't sound related at all. How long has this been affecting you?"

"Pretty much my whole life, but it seems to be getting worse. When I started to walk, I remember my parents saying they were concerned because I would walk on my toes. Which reminds me, now sometimes when I walk people tell me that it looks like I'm limping sometimes, but all my friends say that is my normal walk."

At this point Jessie chimes in, "I wouldn't really say that it's limping, but it looks more like she doesn't want to pick up her feet and they appear to drag a little bit."

"Okay," turning back to me the doctor asks, "Have you seen anyone for this before? And if this has been going on your whole life, why are you just now getting it checked out?"

"My parents told me that they took me to different doctors and even a couple neurologists when I was little, but all of them didn't think anything was wrong with me and told them I would grow out of it."

"Do you have trouble chewing or swallowing?"

"No."

"Does your hand sometimes cramp up and you're not able to move your fingers or return your hand to a normal position?"

"Actually, yes."

"Do you have any numbness or tingling?"

"Not that I have noticed."

"Is there anything else that you can think of that might be related to this?"

"Not that I can think of."

"Okay, I would like you to take off your shoes and socks and sit here," he says opening the door, "I will be back in a minute."

After a brief moment of waiting, Dr. Manteca re-enters the room to see me sitting on the chair he told me to climb onto, with my bare feet dangling down. "I'm going to do some neurological tests which may seem silly, but they will help me to see what we're dealing with." Next, he says, "First I'm going to test your peripheral vision. Look straight at me." He holds his left hand out to my right side holding up four fingers and asks, "How many fingers am I holding up?"

"Four," I reply, wondering if this is what a sobriety test feels like.

Again, holding out three fingers, this time with his right hand on my left side Dr Manteca asks "Now how many?"

"Three," I reply.

"Okay, good. Now I want you to follow my fingers but only with your eyes. Don't move your head at all, keep it still."

I do the best I can, and he tells me to stop moving my head. I am not even aware that my head is moving and have a hard time with this, but we try again. As soon as I focus on not moving my head at all, I can follow his fingers using only my eyes and he tells me I am doing good. Next, he continues to test my reflexes. He takes an anvil and slams it against my left kneecap, "That's interesting, that is a very weak response," after my leg barely jerks. Then he does the same thing to my right leg, "Oh I'm sorry. Too late, you're dead," he jokes since my leg doesn't budge. Next, he tests the reflexes in my feet, but he keeps to himself whether this is a normal reaction or not. After this, the doctor takes a long metal object in the shape of a lollipop with a wooden handle. "Let me know when you stop feeling this," he says as he bangs the metal against the counter before touching the metal to my foot. After a few seconds, "It stopped," I inform, kind of in a question.

"Nope, it's still buzzing pretty hard," The doctor announces before repeating the procedure on my other foot. Again, the same thing happens. Next, he grabs my big toe on my left foot and lifts it up, "This is up, and this is down," as he moves my toe to match his statement. "Now, close your eyes and tell me if it's up or down."

"Good," the neurologist says after a series of ups and downs with my toes. Then he reaches for a safety pin and places the sharp end against the skin of my right foot. "This is sharp," the doctor flips it so the dull side is now touching my skin, "and this is dull. Now close your eyes and tell me if I'm touching you with the sharp side or the dull side."

"Good," the doctor says once again. "Now stand up. I want you to walk from here to the door and back, but instead of your normal walk I want you to walk on your heels."

"Um, okay," I stutter nervously before almost falling over and trying to take a step on my heels. I try again and again, but the entire distance is more like starting with my heels and each step ending with my foot flat against the floor.

"All right, now walk the same place that you just did, but this time, walk on your tippy-toes." This is much easier than walking on my heels, but still a little on the difficult side. However, I am able to keep my balance and complete the exercise this time around.

"Okay, now I would like you to see you walk your normal, everyday walk. Step outside with me," Dr. Manteca insists as he holds the door open. "Just walk your normal walk going down to the end of the hallway and back."

Still barefoot, I do as the doctor says wondering how gross the floor is. He has me walk for him one more time this way and this time I start to wonder how many other people have walked barefoot across this hallway. "Let's go back in here and there's one more thing I would like to see," the neurologist directs again holding the door open. "Now I want you to do a knee-dip for me and you can use the edge of this for support if you need to," pointing to the oddly shaped exam table.

"What do you mean by knee dip," I asked completely confused.

"Squat down as low as you can and stand back up."

Holding onto the edge of the chair I squat down as much as I can before falling over, with my left knee bending a little bit more than my right. Using the strength of my left arm to push myself back up, "Whoa!" I exclaim as I nearly fall over.

"That's weird," the doctor says calmly.

"Yeah," I agree quietly.

"Go ahead and sit back down," After I'm seated the doctor says, "I would like you to have some blood drawn, it's just downstairs to your left and you don't need to fast so you can have that done today. Also, I would like to schedule you for an Electromyogram. My assistant will get you all the information you need and set that up for you. Thank you for coming in, it was nice meeting you. Just wait here and Jenny will be here soon to go over everything with you."

"Okay, thank you. It was nice to meet you too." Almost immediately after Dr. Manteca leaves the room, a young blonde woman walks in, "Hi, I'm Jenny."

"Courtney," I reply a little intimidated, "It's nice to meet you."

"You as well. I understand you need to have an EMG. Do you know what that is?"

"No.

"Okay, it's an electromyography test. More commonly known as an EMG. It measures the conductions in your nerves to see how well they are performing. I will also give you a paper on it." She hands the paper over. "The only restrictions are no lotion and no caffeine beforehand. Your limbs will also need to be warm for the test to work. If you are too cold, we can't do the test because the machine won't measure any of the conductivity so be sure to dress warm that day. Let me see what Dr. Manteca's schedule looks like. How about Wednesday, February 26th at 9:30 am?"

"That works for me, thank you." I write enter the date and time into my phone calendar and imagine what the EMG will feel like.

Chapter 5

Another month of waiting and my appointment for the electromyography is finally here. At my previous appointment the nurse told me to be sure to wear shorts and a tank top, but to make sure I stay bundled up, so my limbs are kept warm. I remember her saying that if my arms or legs or cold they won't be able to do the testing because it will interfere with how the machine works. This morning I am nervous, and I forgot to pick my clothes out last night. My appointment is fairly early in the morning and I have to try and figure out what to wear. My eyes come across a pair of blue gym shorts that were sitting in my laundry basket. Perfect, now all I need is a top! Luckily, I can peer into my drawer where all my tank tops are kept and I pull out a pink one that I recently purchased. The weather is starting to warm up, so I was trying to prepare for summer and purchased the tank top about a week ago. Now, in order to stay warm, I need to wear something over these clothes. "Jeans and a sweatshirt will do," I think to myself as I pull the jeans up over my shorts and zip up a sweatshirt over my tank top. They also had instructed me to not drink caffeine prior to the appointment, because it too would interfere with the machines. This meant skipping my regular cup of coffee this morning, which is no problem since I have been on a break since they had originally scheduled my appointment before they rescheduled it for another two weeks out. This time, Kallie is coming with me to my appointment for emotional support.

Once we arrive, I knew where to go because of how traumatized I was trying to find the place with my last appointment. I check in with the neurology receptionist and sign the paperwork for the consent to perform the test. When the nurse calls me back for the test, Kallie tries to come with me, but the nurse stops her from following us into the room. I am so nervous that I freeze up. Instead of asking the nurse to allow her to come back with me, I am rendered speechless and don't say a word as I follow the nurse into the testing room.

In the exam room, there is a large table and computer with an arm sticking out from it. The arms have needles attached to the ends and the machine looks interesting and scary. At first, the nurse asks me to change into a hospital gown. I absolutely hate hospital gowns, so I inform her about wearing a tank top and shorts under my clothes. She asks, "Are the shorts flexible and loose? Will the doctor be able to move the clothing if necessary?" When I describe the clothing to her she says they will be okay and asks me to change into those. As soon as she leaves the room, I strip off my jacket and pull my jeans off before sitting on the exam table waiting for the doctor. I notice the warmth in the room, but still feel a little chill run through me as I am nervous and not sure what to expect. All my research told me this will be a painful procedure and be extremely uncomfortable.

Finally, the doctor arrives and asks if I am ready to begin. Once Dr. Manteca is inside, he walks me through each step that he will be performing. First, he places electrodes onto my legs. Then he takes out the giant needles. Once he has a needle inserted, he asks me to flex my muscles. This is the part I am most nervous about.

Everything I have read or seen about EMG's say that this is the most painful part of the procedure. The doctor senses my fear and hesitation and says that it will be okay and not too uncomfortable. I do as he says and try my best to flex my muscle. I take a deep breath and am at ease. This is nothing like it was described online and I didn't feel any pain, just an odd sensation. However, the hardest part comes next when he asks me to relax my muscle. I do as he says, or at least I think I relax my muscle, but he continues to tell me to relax my muscle. I eventually have to tell him that I am relaxing my muscle, but he still tells me that I am not. He gently pulls the needle electrode out of my leg and shakes my leg telling it to relax before reinserting into my leg. I guess that worked because he says I am now relaxed. This happens a few more times throughout the test where Dr. Manteca must shake my arm or my leg in order to get my muscle to relax. By the end of the test, I am no longer nervous. I had been so worked up because everything I read previously said the process was more intense and painful. This did not feel painful at all to me. A little uncomfortable sure, but not painful.

In the end, Dr. Manteca tells me he had to send the results for further evaluation, but it looks to him like I have some type of muscular dystrophy. At the mention of muscular dystrophy, so many thoughts are racing through my mind. In all my research throughout high school trying to figure out what might be wrong with me, I kept coming back to muscular dystrophy. However, I also thought it was most likely to occur in males and I am a girl. I am also scared and don't know what that means for my future, other than I will most likely never be able to do lunges or stand up from the ground without using my hands, the only things that I have ever really wanted to be able to do. My mind wondered if I might still be able to work towards running a full mile one day. Dr. Manteca pulls me back to reality and tells me that he knows it is scary, takes my arm, and tells me that everything will be okay. It's almost as if he had read my thoughts. Tears are starting to form in the corner of my eyes as so many thoughts are firing through my brain. It takes all my energy not to let them fall. In that moment a million thoughts are coming to me; I finally have a diagnosis, something I can finally use to explain to others what is going on with me, I finally know that this is real and I'm really not lazy like so many people have assumed. I also start to question what my life will look like in the future and I wonder how no one else could have noticed this when muscular dystrophy seems to be a childhood disease. I also wonder what my life would have been like if I actually had been diagnosed all those years ago when my parents first started looking for answers. He continues to tell me that he doesn't think there is anything with my nerves and that is a good sign since things get much worse once the nerves are involved. He tells me that my case is now out of his hands and he is sending me to a specialist that will know more about my situation. He hands me a card to the Muscular Dystrophy Association clinic and tells me to set up an appointment. He tells me to call them right away to set up an appointment and not wait for them to call me. Again, he tells me that everything will be okay, and they will take good care of me.

Once I walk out of the office I barely glance at Kallie and she can immediately see that something is wrong. She follows me into the elevator and asks what they had said. Through deep breaths and holding back tears I tell her everything. Once we get to my car, she hugs me and tells me to take my time now that the tears are starting to fall.

She also tells me that the doctor telling me that everything will be okay is a good sign and to wait and see what the other place has to say. Then she suggests I call the number on the MDA card now to set up the appointment and get a step ahead, before jumping to any conclusions.

I immediately call and set up an appointment with the MDA clinic, but the only appointment they have available is for the end of March. I take the appointment and once I am ready Kallie and I continue to a shopping adventure and to eat.

*   *   *   *   *

The next month leads to a series of bouts of depression and things I can't even remember now. I was starting to fall into some bad habits and going out and drinking a lot. On top of all the emotions I was feeling from the recent diagnosis, my friendship group was having problems. It had apparently all started at that New Year's party. Jessie started dating a guy that Kallie was interested in and I had no clue what was happening because I was wrapped up in my own journey. Eventually, Kallie and Jessie quit talking and Daisy took Kallie's side and avoided Jessie as well. I was caught in the middle and told my friends the truth, I thought they were all dumb for fighting over a guy and should not let it come between their friendship.

Things were good for a while, but eventually, Kallie met someone too. Kallie was living with me and my parents at the time and my parents are extremely strict when it comes to guys. They don't allow people to spend the night and my mom caught Kallie's boyfriend leaving one morning. This caused my mom to kick her out of my house and we haven't talked since. Not long after I received a Facebook message from Daisy saying that she didn't know I was such a different person than she thought, and she couldn't trust me, and she couldn't be friends with me anymore. As much as it hurt, I told her I felt the same way and that if she couldn't even hear me out to not come crying back to me when the truth comes out. During the hardest time in my life going through the diagnosis process, I also lost two of my closest, long-time friends. When I needed people to lean on the most, I felt completely abandoned.

 Nothing could have prepared me for what was coming next. The bill I received for the EMG later turned out to be $2000. The bill for the neurology appointment itself was $700 and the blood draw was $200. For the cost of care, I decided to go onto my parent's insurance with Kaiser in April, when it was time for an open enrollment period again to help keep the costs of the medical bills down. I know I am jumping ahead a little bit here, but it's all part of the story, and this is the best place to put it. The bill from the MDA clinic was also $500 and now I am owing $3000 in medical bills on a part-time retail income. As they say, when it rains, it pours.

Chapter 6

Here we are on a rainy March morning in the foggy city of San Francisco. No matter how much I tried to keep everything to myself and how much I didn't want to share what was going on with me with my family, my mom was now fully aware of my entire medical situation. She insists on going with me and puts a guilt trip on me when I suggest that I don't need her to come with me. It's not that I didn't want her there, but at the same time I felt like I would be holding information back because I didn't want to hurt her feelings if she is with me and I have to say the reason I waited so long to say anything is because I felt like I had to keep it a secret and keep everything hidden inside.

 In the end, my mom is the one to go with me to my appointment at the Muscular Dystrophy Association clinic, instead of going with one of my friends or by myself like I had originally planned. As I'm still trying to cope with the loss of my friends from earlier in the year, I am happy to have another person in my corner. As nervous as I am about opening up in front of my mom, at least I don't have to drive this way. I'm nervous about sharing why I waited so long to get checked out with the doctor in front of my mom mainly because she is the reason that I have waited so long to ask what is wrong with me. Her not talking about my condition with me and only sometimes telling my brother that she didn't think I was capable of doing some things is what led me to be completely closed off to myself and the rest of the world. Growing up that way, I felt like I needed to keep my true self completely hidden and like I was damaged goods. I don't want her to feel like she did the wrong thing by not talking about my muscle weakness with me because I understand her reasons for not wanting me to feel like there was something wrong with me. However, I also had my own feelings that had already formed and telling the truth about them to get to the bottom of everything would mean that if she was with me, she would hear my side of things and most likely get upset. The doctors had started to tell her she was crazy when she originally tried to talk to them about my condition when I first started walking and she didn't want me to feel like it was a problem for me. However, this is what made me feel self-conscious and afraid to speak up about my condition. As we drive into the parking lot, we find a place to park and begin walking towards the clinic. The entire direction is uphill, not fun more someone with a muscle problem in their legs. Not only that, but I was walking at my pace to keep up the momentum to get up that hill and in doing so, I was ahead of my mom. Because of the pace gap, she started saying that I should slow down and wait for her. In my mind, I was only doing what I could to make it to the clinic.

Once we get to the front doors I am out of breath and tired out. I'm not sure I should be at this place as the sign on the door reads MDA/ALS clinic. Knowing that the first doctor I saw regarding this issue mentioned I could have early onset ALS, seeing the letters on the sign did not put me at ease. Upon arriving, I check-in at the front desk and inform them I have an appointment. They tell me to have a seat and ask if I would like some water. "No, thank you" is all I can say. I am so nervous; I just want this day to be over with. I want an answer to what I have been experiencing and I am closer than ever to finally receiving one. I look around in the waiting room, watching people come and go. Everyone that is coming in is either a young child or an older person. Most people are using a cane or are in a wheelchair. Again, I question whether I should be here, as I have not seen anyone at all that looks like me. After all, the first doctor did mention that I could have early onset ALS, but the second doctor was convinced otherwise. I am scared and feel alone even though I have so many people that care about me now and that are supportive of me in this new chapter of my life. I feel like I am completely misplaced and somehow my "newfound" life is not meant for me, but for someone else. I start thinking about what could happen and how much my life would change if I needed to start using a cane or a walker, or even worse, a wheelchair, like everyone else in this place seems to need. I am so independent right now and can't even begin to imagine how everything would have to change if I need to start using any of these devices.

My anxious thoughts are broken when I hear a voice call my name. I'm wearing blue jeans and a long sleeve t-shirt, my usual dress attire, and it's keeping me warm in the rainy weather. Monica introduces herself and calls me back after what seems like forever in the waiting room pondering a completely different life; one I never want to live. I go into the room and immediately Monica wraps the blue cuff around my arm to take my blood pressure and temperature. The blood pressure machine is automatic, and it can't find my pressure on the first try so it continues to squeeze my arm and loosen as I try not to cry from all the uneasiness, I am facing combined with the pain of the machine. She asks if this is my first time here in which I reply, "Yes, I was referred because the neurologist I recently saw thinks I have some kind of muscular dystrophy."

"Okay, yes, I see the referral," she hesitates, "We will take care of you. You are in great hands with Dr. Calico and he will be right in."

Monica leaves the room and leaves my mom and I waiting once again. My mom awkwardly smiles at me, trying to give me some comfort, which only makes me feel more awkward. She has done this at every single appointment I have ever been to and even though it's meant to be a gesture of comfort, it makes me uneasy. I feel like there is something unspoken in her face that she won't say, and I haven't been able to crack the code. This room is larger than any other doctor's office I have been in. There is the usual long table and the chair next to the exam table, but also a lot of space. After only a few minutes a middle-aged man with a bald head and blue eyes enters the room, "Hello, I am Dr. Calico. I have looked over your referral. I see here some things that you have concerns about. What is going on? I would like to hear it from you."

I explain, "I have been tripping and falling a lot." I describe how I started at my primary physician's office and explain about being referred to a neurologist. Next, I tell the specialist about my encounter with Dr. Manteca and all about the EMG and how he thinks I have some type of muscular dystrophy, but how he didn't know much about it and thought I should be referred to a specialist."

"Okay," Dr. Calico says questioning, "How long has this been going on?"

I tell him about walking on my toes when I was a baby and constantly falling. My mom jumps in and talks about how she took me to several different doctors when I was little and how each and every one of those doctors told her that it was a phase I was going through and something I would eventually grow out of. By the way, I never did. When the questions were coming, having my mom there to help answer the questions that I couldn't and fill in gaps was really comforting. In the end, I'm glad she came. Anyway, I talk about my recent falls at work and how I'm not gaining any strength even though I am working out at least four times per week and doing everything I have learned to try and increase my muscle tone.

The doctor then asks the question I didn't want to answer in front of my mom, "Why are you choosing to see someone about this now?"

I again explain myself, "I want to know if I am able to have kids and if this is something that I would pass on to my kids. Also, I have always wondered, and other people are questioning what is wrong with me as well." Something I didn't mention was how I struggled with wanting to know my whole life but thinking that I needed to hide from my own body. I don't think it would have mattered either. Although, I do sometimes wonder if they would have come to an accurate diagnosis sooner if they knew all of my reasoning for waiting. I also wonder if they would have referred me to a psychologist instead of assuming that I was fine. I didn't want my mom to feel bad for making me feel like I couldn't talk about it and what was I supposed to say? After all, she is sitting right next to me and I have a long ride home with her. I didn't want her to question me about it in the car. I just want this day to be over with and to find out what I have so I can get better and move on with my life. However, in the end, I am really glad she came with me and I am happy to have her on my side being super supportive.

The specialist nods his head in an understanding way and asks me to perform some tasks. Again, I am asked to walk on my toes and my heels. Also, to walk normally. I have to demonstrate how I get up from a chair. Then the doctor asks how I get up from the floor. Something no one has ever asked me before, so I offer to demonstrate. I sit down on the cold; hard floor and I first go to my knees. Then all in one motion I push myself up into a push-up position. Next, I stick my butt into the air, moving my left leg closer to my hands, then my right. As I'm moving my right leg towards my palms, I'm starting to come to a standing position. In order to maintain my balance, I push my hands against my quadriceps as I pull myself into a standing position. I also have to demonstrate several strength tests, a few of which I fail as I can't move my legs at all. For example, Dr. Calico has me do all of the same tests from my original appointment and the previous neurologist. In addition, he has me lift my leg straight up from a sitting position. On my right side, I can't get it to lift at all. On my left, I can lift my leg, but only a little bit. The doctor keeps saying, "Hmmm" and "That's interesting" throughout the entire exam. I don't know what he is thinking, and I don't know what to think myself. Finally, at the end of the exam, he tells me he thinks I have Limb-Girdle Muscular Dystrophy, Type 2A. I have absolutely no idea what that means, but finally, I have an answer! An answer I had been waiting for my entire life! All I need is a blood test to confirm it.

I ask what Limb-Girdle Muscular Dystrophy is and what the Type 2A means, but as the doctor is explaining it, all I hear is that it is a rare disease, I will not be able to get stronger, and I will eventually need to use a walking aid. The doctor tells me that I have a very good prognosis and asks what I am doing for work right now and if I am going to school. When I tell him retail for work, he tells me that I should find a different line of work. Then when I tell him that I just finished my AA degree in psychology, already have an AA in humanities, and am working on a medical billing and coding certificate, before working on becoming a sign language interpreter he seems to only hear the first thing and tells me that I should stick with psychology as it is the perfect line of work, sitting and talking to people all day. I fail to mention that the psychology degree is supposed to be a temporary filler until I can finish my sign language interpreting certificate and continue to become a nursing student. With the news, I feel like the dreams of my future are crushed and nursing can no longer be in my future.

Dr. Calico starts to schedule this blood test, but when I ask, he tells me I won't be able to get in for the blood test and another appointment before April. At this point, my heart sinks. I am so close to knowing for sure exactly what has been going on inside my body, but at the same time, so far away. My health insurance is switching to Kaiser in April, and I won't be able to go see the MDA doctor once my insurance switches. I don't know what to do at this moment. I explain the insurance situation to him, and he suggests I set up an appointment with Kaiser as soon as my insurance kicks in and request to see a neurologist with them. The doctor gives me the results from the EMG and his findings and tells me to take them with me to Kaiser. He tells me to explain everything to them and all they will need to do is a blood test to confirm the diagnosis. Thinking I only needed a blood test was okay. But here we are, the beginning of March, and yet again, I have to wait a

month to figure anything out and receive confirmation of
my disease.

Chapter 7

April finally rolls around and finally I am at a point where I can schedule an appointment with a new provider inside of an unfamiliar insurance policy and start the process all over again. It's a good thing I did too! A couple weeks after setting up the next appointment I receive a bill in the mail from the original neurologist and the MDA clinic. My total medical costs for this year are already upwards of $3000. I work a part-time job at a major retail chain making $12 per hour. How in the world am I supposed to pay the high cost of medical bills on that income and be paying for my schooling all at the same time? I can't afford to have a disease or anything wrong with me, I can't afford to be taking so much time off work, and now I'm wishing even more so that I had have questioned things when I was younger. During this time, I am also enrolled in a medical billing and coding certificate program as I am trying to find a job with flexible hours before trying to resume a nursing program and I am paying for everything completely on my own. At this point, I feel like I'll never be able to get out of debt and never be able to move out of my parents' house.

Now I'm sitting at my first appointment in an office out of town because the last thing I want is for anyone that I know to see me and ask about why I am here. I'm sitting in the waiting room counting the squares on the ceiling trying to keep my mind off things when someone walks up to me and says, "Courtney? It's nice to meet you, come on back." Like every other appointment, they take my vitals, ask why I'm here, then tell me the doctor will be in in a minute.

Pretty soon the doctor walks in an introduces himself, "Hi, I'm Dr. Mel."

"Nice to meet you, I'm Courtney," I sheepishly reply as I hand him my EMG results and explain that my insurance had just switched before they were able to confirm anything. Next, I find myself explaining everything I had gone through from starting the process with my primary care doctor, to seeing Dr. Manteca, and then most recently the MDA clinic and Dr. Calico. I explain about the notes from the MDA clinic and how Dr. Calico thought I had Limb-Girdle Muscular Dystrophy, Type 2A. The new physician takes the information and looks over all of the documentation. After about two minutes (it feels more like 20) of sitting in silence, I'm holding my breath when the doctor finally says he still wants to examine me.

Again, I am asked to walk my normal walk, walk on my toes, and attempt to walk on my heels across the room. Once again, I try to lift my leg while in a sitting position, which this time I can't do at all. And again, I need to extend my leg up while I'm in a sitting position while the doctor tries to push down. This time, the doctor asks me to just try extending my legs as far out as they will go, which I can't even get parallel to the floor. The next thing this doctor says to me is something I will never forget. He says, "Wow! Your legs are extremely weak. It's amazing you're able to walk!" Then, with a sorrowful look in his eyes, he tells me he is going to refer me to a neurologist to get the testing started right away. He follows up and says that with LGMD there is a normal life expectancy into my 70s, but they can't be sure until they have a confirmed diagnosis. He also tells me he wants me to see a physical therapist and tells me to give them a call right away to set up an appointment.

At this point, the appointment concludes with Dr. Mel telling me to take another blood test, but it was not the same one to determine a LGMD diagnosis. Instead, it was the one for determining my creatine kinase levels, something else I had already done. The doctor tells me it is urgent that I get in with the neurologist and sets up the appointment for me without allowing me the two weeks I need to properly request the time off work. Since I am here anyway, I go to the lab and have them complete the blood test. Once I return to my car, I call and try to set up the appointment with the physical therapist. The lady on the phone asks me who I would like to see, and not knowing who anyone is at this location, I tell her I have absolutely no idea. She recommends someone for me, but I am not able to get in for an appointment right away, so she schedules one in the future for me.

Now, I am really scared and am not sure what to do or what to think. How can I have gone on for so long with such limited strength that I shouldn't be able to walk now? I am so independent; how can I handle not being able to walk? This is also the first time I ever heard the term, "life expectancy," how long they expect me to live. They told me my life expectancy was a normal lifespan most likely into my 70s, but they didn't know how much longer I would be able to walk without a walking aid of some kind. My next neurology appointment takes place in a week, but it feels like an eternity while I am waiting with all of this new-found information on my mind to ponder. I almost want to give up right now, but I decided to keep going because I feel like I am so close to finally receiving an answer I have been waiting for my entire life.

Chapter 8

Here I am now, phase two of my restart journey.
Once again, I'm sitting in a waiting room of a neurology
office wondering what is going on and wondering what will
become of my life. I guess this is starting to feel like my
new normal now, something I should be getting used to.
Again, I start to question if I really want to continue with
this process and getting diagnosed, but I'm already in the
office and it's too late to back out now.

"Courtney…" a woman's voice interrupts my
thoughts. It is the nurse calling me back. By this time, I
have learned to dress in shorts and a tank top for my
appointments to avoid having to change into a hospital
gown. It is the start of spring and this dress attire is
appropriate with the warmth of the sun, but in the
mornings, everything is chilly outside, so I am also wearing
a sweater. I take off my jacket and start to wonder, "What
will become of me and my life? 23-years-old and I'm told I
should not be able to walk."

Finally, the new neurologist knocks on the door,
"Good morning! I'm Dr. Fauva." She extends her hand out
to me for a handshake.

"Good morning," I greet with a blank smile as I
return the shake.

"Wow, you have a strong handshake," she exclaims
before quickly moving on, "I have reviewed your notes and
I would like to do an exam if that's all right?"

At this point, I ask about the blood test for LGMD. The doctor dismisses my request, "Let's get started. First, will you walk for me?"

I stand up and repeat the tasks from all of my previous appointments. Again, walking across the cold hardwood floor barefoot on my heels and my toes. Then the muscle strength routine as this unfamiliar stranger pushes down against my skin with a few repeat exercises. The same results every time and the same familiar grunts and groans. This time, something new happens as well. The physician asks, "Will you please smile for me?" I do so again and again, and she comments, "You have a beautiful, crooked smile. Can you smile wider?" Next, she has me do different things with my face. Once these exercises come to an end, she tells me to take a seat.

"Based on your smile, the unevenness and the way your right side is weaker than your left, I'd say you have a mild form of cerebral palsy."

"Okay," I say, here we are again, a different diagnosis and no confirmation.

"I would like you to have a muscle biopsy to look for any atrophy within your muscle and I would also like for you to start physical therapy. I am also going to refer you to another neurologist that specializes in muscle disorders."

"Okay," I acknowledge a little confused. I think to myself that I thought I was sent to someone that specializes in muscle disorders, "How soon will you do a muscle biopsy?"

The physician schedules the day of the biopsy for a week from today and also gives me the number to call and set up an appointment with a physical therapist. I am nervous about this because now I need to tell my manager at work what is going on since I am scheduled to work the day of the biopsy. I don't know if they will be okay with me taking the time off, and I haven't even told anyone outside of my immediate family or outside of my friends what has been going on with me. I don't want the whole world to know until I know what's going on. But I need to be responsible and continue to work as well. I even had asked about work and they told me this is important and doesn't allow me to schedule the time in advance and that I will only need to take the rest of the day after the biopsy off and can return to work the next day.

As soon as I return home that day, I call to set up the physical therapy appointment. The operator on the phone asks me who I want to see and not knowing that I was supposed to pick out my own physical therapist before calling, I hadn't even gone online to see who was available. I explain my predicament to the person on the other end of the phone and she suggests I see Kyle and says that he will be great.

"That works," I say, "Thank you." And I set up the appointment for a couple days after the muscle biopsy as that was all they had available. Here we are, back to waiting again.

*   *   *   *

The next day when I show up to work, I am completely consumed with anxiety. I am not ready to tell anyone what is going on with me, but I don't feel like I have a choice now. After all, my manager had been asking me almost every day for the past couple of months if everything was okay with me. He knew from January that it wasn't, but I never said anything about what was going on. Now, it is time for me to speak up.

The workday was busy as usual and even though I knew it wasn't the three weeks in advance I needed to request time off, I tried to put the request in the computer. However, because the schedule had already been made, it would not let me. When the manager finally came around to see how everything was going, I think he sensed the anxiety in me because he asked me how things were going for me. This time around, I asked him if I could talk to him. Because things were so busy, he told me to come find him at the end of my shift, which is exactly what I did.

Once my shift ended and I clocked out for the day I found him and asked to talk to him privately. He took me into the back room, and I started to explain everything that had been going on. I didn't know what to say, and I didn't know how to handle the situation, and I didn't want him or anyone to think that I had been dishonest when I had applied and stated on the application that there was nothing wrong with me. So, all I said was that I have some kind of muscular dystrophy. He asked what it is, and not really knowing myself, I described my symptoms. Then I went on to explain all of the tests they had already done and everything they still wanted to do. Then I explained about the muscle biopsy and how they wouldn't let me schedule it in advance and asked if I would be able to leave an hour early that day. I also stated that I might need more time off for appointments too. He then told me to let him know what I needed and if there was anything he could do.

I felt a lot better once I finally told someone what was going on, because now I didn't feel like I was carrying around a big secret everywhere I went. Looking back on it now, I think I probably would have had a lot more support if I didn't feel so ashamed of myself and had just shared what was going on with me. However, I also didn't want to seem like someone that just complains, especially if it turned out nothing was going on with me, like all the doctors from my childhood had agreed on.

Chapter 9

This April morning starts out just like any other spring morning. I work at a retail store in the early morning hours, only this time, I have to ask to leave early for my biopsy appointment. I feel so much anxiety as I'm asking to leave, and everyone comments on me leaving early. I still haven't shared with many people because I don't want everyone to know. Luckily, they let me go. Again, I wasn't given the choice to ask for the time off, which I was already annoyed with the medical facility for.

During the pre-operation period, they inform me to take it easy for the rest of the day, but I was fine to be out and about. They also tell me I should have no problem returning to work the next day and resuming my normal duties even as physical as they are. I even point out that I am on my feet for my entire shift and ask if that will be a problem and they proceed to tell me I will be fine, but they'll give me a note to take to work for today.

Since my mom knows all about what was going on with me at this point, she insists on taking the time off and coming with me to my appointment. They previously told me I would be able to drive after the procedure; however, they are biopsying my right leg, my driving leg. My mom drives me to the appointment this morning and in my head, I am questioning everything the doctors have told me this far. I am also very nervous as I spent last night reading all about muscle biopsies and how much pain they cause.

As I arrive, they immediately take me back into an exam room. They explain the procedure and any risks associated. I sign the papers without thinking twice, somewhat now of a routine. It's not like I have a choice anyway if I want them to continue finding out what is wrong with me. I had also previously been studying to be a nurse before my life threw me some major curveballs. I know all the risks are unlikely and everything has to be included just in case something does go wrong. My hands are shaking as I sign and date for a procedure, I have no idea what to expect.

Previously, I had looked online and everywhere I searched made a muscle biopsy out to be a big deal. Every website I landed on said it was a painful procedure; however, I read the same thing about the EMG before going in and that was no big deal. All of the websites also said that with a muscle biopsy a rest period from anything physical would be required for a week. When I looked up a muscle biopsy online, I thought the internet was exaggerating like it does with most things.

After the authorization papers are signed a doctor comes in with a couple of other people. All of them have horrifying looks on their faces. I study each and every one of them all insinuating that something was terribly wrong. I stay silent and realize at this moment that these are the people who will be operating on me and I realize the fear comes from how they are perceiving my current condition. It is that same look the prior neurologist provided and before her, the same look from the physician whom I first presented my situation with Kaiser. This makes me feel even more uneasy and I start to shake again. This entire time I am trying to hide how scared and nervous I feel and am doing everything I can to not break down crying.

Finally, after what seems like forever the surgeon breaks the silence, "Hello there." I am Dr. Rose and I will be performing the biopsy today. This is Brad and he is a medical student. Is it okay if he helps me out today?"

"Sure," I give my permission, not realizing what I was getting into. "How else are medical students supposed to learn," I wondered to myself also thinking that if I was a medical student I would hope the patients would say the same thing for me.

They start by rubbing a numbing cream on my leg before giving me a shot of lidocaine to numb the area of my right quadricep. At first everything is fine and painless, then the make the incision. At this point I am feeling something poking me and I mention it to the staff in the room. They tell me that even though I am numb, I would still be able to feel some things against my skin. For now, the pain isn't too unbearable, so I leave it alone. Gradually I feel them going in deeper and deeper until I can't take it anymore.

"Ouch!" I cried, "I don't think I am numb! I feel something is stabbing the inside of my leg."

The doctor gives me a cold look, "Courtney, we can not give you any more anesthesia. This is all we can do. You will be feeling some things because of the muscle tissue." The tone of her voice annoys me, and I am stuck with nothing else to say. They have all the power as I am lying here helpless on this table, being stabbed by someone that wants to be digging in.

Tears start to roll down my face and I started gasping in pain. Finally, I am able to turn gasps into deep breaths, anything I can do to keep from screaming and scaring everyone in this room. After all, they are literally stabbing deep into my leg at this point and all I can do is lie there helplessly, trying to keep still in order to avoid any more pain, not that any more pain would have been possible or noticeable.

Finally, they tell me, "We are almost done, but we do see some atrophying. We are going to take out some of the muscle and send it away for confirmation."

"It's not like the pain can become any worse," I think as I try to form the words to say that would be okay. Man was I wrong! They cut in even deeper than before and I can feel the tearing of the muscle where they decide to slice into. I guess they think weakness means numbness because they kept asking me, but weakness does not mean numbness and I can no longer hold in my screams. I feel the procedure will never end, but at least now the worst part is over. At least that's what I think and the same thing I hear is a faint, muffled sound behind the pain that is blocking my mental clarity.

Finally, the doctor queries, "We are ready to close. Will it be okay to let Brad close doing the sutures?"

"Okay," I agree. The only words I can force out after the previous events. I've had stitches before and it's not like the pain from the stitches would even compare to the pain from having part of my muscle ripped out. Again, stitches are like sewing, so how could a med student do any worse than someone with lots of practice?

Wrong again. Brad starts out okay, but the further we go, the more I feel. I can feel every poke of the needle, every in and every out. By the time the procedure finishes, my leg is completely numb from the pain and I finally hear the words, "We're done" and "you did great" at the end of a very dark and long tunnel. They roll me back into an exam room and go over when to call if I experience any severe side effects, like red skin surrounding the wound or pus leaking out. Eventually the time comes when they tell me I can get dressed and am free to leave. My mom hands me my clothes and I put my shirt on first as that is easiest for me. Then I attempt to put yoga pants on. A square of gauze lies across the top of the wound from where they did the biopsy, covered with medical tape, but I am still concerned about the material. I first put my left leg into the pant leg, followed by the right, which I have to lift up to put into my pant leg. Then I slowly stand up and pull the pants up over me and over my leg, being careful and trying to not touch the material to the gauze.

At least I am no longer under the knife and am free from being stabbed any longer. Unfortunately, I was gifted an immense, throbbing pain that will not recede no matter what I try. They inform me I will be okay, and it shouldn't hurt for more than a few days. They tell me I will be fine to return to work the next day. At the current state I am in I don't even know if I'll be able to walk, let alone be lifting heavy items at a timed pace. I decide to eat something once I return home, even though the pain is so great I am not sure if I will even be able to eat anything.

On the way home, I can feel every single bump in the road, and it hurts like a truck is running over my leg every time. Once we finally arrive home, I am able to keep everything down and I relax and watch TV keeping my leg positioned on the couch. By 7 pm I am still in a tremendous amount of pain. I don't think I will be able to move the next day so I e-mail my manager and state the amount of pain I am currently facing from the earlier procedure and state that I am not sure if I will be able to make it into work the next morning.

Later, I receive a reply to come in anyway and if it was still too much pain to ask to leave early. I set my alarm for the appropriate time in the middle of the night to ensure I will be giving myself plenty of time to make it into work the next day. After all, I feel like I can't call in sick now. I already pretty much mentioned I would be doing just that, and my request had been denied.

When my alarm sounds in the morning, I don't need to wake up. I have been hurting all night long. I force myself out of my bed and onto my feet. My hands are trembling as I try to make my way through my room to grab my clothes for today. I grab the clothes and hobble downstairs to the shower. Here comes the most challenging part of my morning routine. My wound can't get wet, but my hair is a mess. If I don't wash it, it will turn into a grease fest like the times I didn't have time to shower in the past. In order to show up to my job in a presentable manner, I let down the showerhead and turn the water on. I hurdle the upper part of my body over the bathtub and rinsed my hair with the flexibility the showerhead offers. This is a challenge as the wound on my leg bumps the outer side of the tub a couple times, causing me to let out a sigh of pain. A 15-minute task is taking twice as long with my new leg accessory. The entire routine takes longer than expected, but luckily, I am able to leave for work at my usual time.

Upon arrival, I limp to the front doors. No one asks why I was limping, maybe it isn't as obvious as I thought. The day continues just like any other, I clock in and they send me to work in the back to help with unloading the truck. I do the best I can trying to avoid scraping my leg against the metal. This task is successful until towards the end of the unloading process when I bang my wound right against the metal, I am standing next to. "Ugh!" I let out and take a deep breath trying to keep my cool and not show how much excruciating pain I am in. I guess I did a good job of hiding it because soon enough we were done and given our assignments for the day without anyone asking me what is wrong.

My assignment is to work in a group, like the majority of the team. A couple of people were given separate assignments, but nothing out of the ordinary. Here I am trying to keep up the pace hurt and all and not reveal to anyone that I am struggling or in excruciating pain. A couple of people do eventually ask why I am limping, but I tell them all I have a cut on my leg, nothing from the truth. I keep ignoring all the signs that are telling me to stop and rest my leg and instead I keep pushing through. A few times the manager kept telling me I needed to pick up the pace; I guess I was performing at a slower rate than normal.

Finally, they call for a break and there is only an hour left in that shift. I feel like even an hour will drag on forever and I need something up to help me manage to get through the rest of the shift. Luckily, I am at a store and anything I need is just a purchase away. I decide on ibuprofen, a healthy, Hershey bar snack, and a coke to wash it down. When they ring me up, they ask if I am okay and I simply state that my leg is hurting. I make it through the rest of the shift and the drive home and rest for the rest of the day.

The next week pretty much mimicked that day. I was taking ibuprofen to manage the pain and I did so without a break between any doses. My stomach started to hurt, but I ignored it. The pain in my leg was much worse than an unsettling stomach. Finally, the time came where I could get through the week, still in pain, but without the aid of medicine My stomach returned to its normal state and life continued to go on.

Chapter 10

Two days after my muscle biopsy, I am sitting in another waiting room in a medical office. This time, the appointment is to be evaluated by a physical therapist and to see what they might be able to do to help me. I am not sure what to expect, so I arrive at the office 15 minutes early to fill out the paperwork and get things rolling. I am seeing Brian for the first time, as the lady on the phone had suggested.

The paperwork is asking all of the usual questions that a first-time patient form will ask. However, I am having a really hard time filling it out. The first question asks about where the problem is, so I am easily able to state in my legs and circle the right quadricep where it asks me to circle the area on my body. However, the next question I stumble on. It is asking what caused my problem and when it started. I only have a tiny line to write on and not being sure what to put on this line I write muscle problem and several years ago. As I continue the questions seem to get harder and I'm unsure how to answer them. Jessie tells me to just leave it be for now and explain the answers to the physical therapist. That's what I do and wait again.

As we are waiting in the waiting room, I take a look around and observe everyone else that is sitting near us. There isn't anyone else our age around and everyone is older. Some are using canes, some in wheelchairs, but most are walking at a slow pace with silver strands ling their heads. Their son or daughter is with them and the son/daughter appears to even be doubled my age. Again, I am feeling like I don't belong, and I start to question how things will go.

Several people are coming in and out from beige double doors in the right-hand corner of the waiting room and going up to a patient and bringing them back through the doors with them. Time and time again this is happening, but none of them are Brian. I keep glancing at my watch because I am already nervous, and this is something I do when nervous. Thirty minutes have passed since my appointment was supposed to be scheduled and I am still wondering if I was somehow misplaced somewhere that I don't belong. Luckily, Jessie is helping to keep my calm and although I am shaky, I am doing okay. Finally, a man wearing a striped polo shirt walks out from behind the double doors, walks over to me and introduces himself. I shake his hand and introduce myself and Jessie and he tells us to follow him back. As I'm standing up, I notice that he is observing exactly how I am pressing on the sides of the chair with my arms to rise to a standing position. Once I am up, I notice that we are about the same height and how he had been watching how I stood up. He opens the double doors and says, "After you." I go through the doors to see a long hallway, from which Brian leads the rest of the way into an oversized waiting room.

Once we are in the exam room, he tells me, "Have a seat" and gestures to the exam table. My friend sits in one of the regular chairs that are also in the room. Brian says he notices how I was walking it looked a little off and he asked if I have always walked this way. At this point, I explain that I don't really know as I don't notice how I walk, and I let Jessie explain what she has seen and how I look like I am limping when I get tired. As a matter of fact, a few years ago I was walking near a hospital with some friends in search of my car and a random person came up to us and gave us unsolicited directions to the emergency room because of the way I was walking. Next, he turns back to me and asks me, "Why are you here?"

I explain about the diagnosis process that I have been through and how I have officially been diagnosed with a type of muscular dystrophy, but they are awaiting the results to see exactly what it is. Then I explain my entire life leading up to this moment, how I was always the last one when running, how I would get out of breath quickly, how I couldn't get up from the ground or anything without using my hands to push up, and about how I did martial arts, played softball, soccer, and basketball when I was younger. I also explained about my legs being extremely weak and expressed concern about my abdominal muscles being weak too.

At this point, Brian started the exam. I had to push my head back and forth while he pushed against it. I had to put my arms together and push and pull. Same with the wrists. All of these being completely normal results. Then came my legs. First, he asked me to lift my knee while it was parallel to the ground. As usual, I couldn't get it up at all on the right side. He kept telling me whenever you are ready, and I had to keep telling him that I was trying. Finally, he said ok and moved on to having me straighten my legs out by extending my knee. On my left, this was okay, but it fell right back down as soon as he touched my leg to try and push against it. Then he had me do the same on the right. This time, I could not get my leg to straighten all the way out. Same as with every other test any medical professional has done. He also tells me that it is amazing how my other muscles have compensated for my weaker muscles and how it is amazing that I can walk still. He mentions braces for my feet to correct the way I walk, but he also said he doesn't think he wants to do that, because that would take walking away from me. After these, he said he sees what the problem is and started showing me some strengthening exercises for me to do. At the end, he asked if I had any questions, and I asked about strengthening my abdominals too. He said for now, he was concerned about my quadriceps and that he wanted to focus on getting those stronger.

First, he shows me the dreaded leg lifts. He has me lie down and bend one knee while trying to keep the other one straight and raise it. My leg barely comes off the table and he says, "So that's a tough one for you then. Hmm, let me think." Next, he puts a foam roller under my knee and has me try to straighten my leg. This I am able to do, but barely. He tells me that this will be one of my exercises and to try and hold the straightened position for 5 seconds every time. Then he has me do bridges, which I can do with ease. Finally, he shows me some stretches to do before sending me on my way.

Chapter 11

Three weeks have now gone by and I haven't heard anything, not one word from the neurologist or anyone else on my care team. Curiosity has gotten the best of me, so I give in and e-mail the neurologist asking if the results have come in yet. Before the procedure she said the results take about two weeks because of having to mail them to the lab and having the results mailed back.

A couple days pass without any response and my anxiety is becoming worse and again I start to wonder if this is really something I want to know. An e-mail finally comes in saying she is going to set up a time to give me a call. "Great!" I think. A phone call from a doctor usually means it's nothing too serious and once I know I can go on to fixing the problem. Maybe all the other doctors jumped ahead to conclusions in their head and all the sorrowful looks were for no reason. My mind was at ease, but the more time that is passing before receiving a phone call from the doctor, the more anxious I am growing.

At the time I thought that time meant she would call when she had time available. I am still waiting and continue to wait, jumping at the phone any time it rings. Finally, an e-mail comes through one day saying I have a phone appointment scheduled with this doctor. Finally, I thought. I was so nervous the day of the phone appointment. I didn't want to go anywhere and do anything and risk missing that call.

In the late afternoon my phone finally rings, "Hello," I answer.

"Hi, is this Courtney? This is Dr. Lian. How are you?"

"Good, thank you. Did the results come in yet from the muscle biopsy?"

"Yes, that is why I am calling. As it turns out, you have Spinal Muscular Atrophy and I'm going to make an educated guess that it's type 3 based on what you told us about your symptoms starting in childhood." The doctor sounds disappointed.

"Okay, great!" I say innocently, "I have never heard of that. What is that, what does it mean, and what are the next steps?" I had no idea what kind of loaded questions those were and I definitely wasn't ready for the answer.

On the other end of the phone, I heard her say, "It's a neuromuscular disease that affects the anterior horn cells. Your motor neurons die off and it's a progressive disease. As the disease continues to progress you will lose the ability to walk, to move your arms, until eventually you become paralyzed…" She kept talking, but I didn't hear another word of what was being said. Here I was, completely confused and focused on one day losing the ability to walk and then thinking about not being able to move at all. How could I even hear anything else? Then I heard her ask, "What's going through your mind right now?"

The question brought me out of the deep trance I had fallen into and suddenly I was at a loss for words. All I could ask was, "If I have kids, will they be affected in the same way as me?" The news kept getting worse as they told me if I had kids it would depend on if the dad was a carrier and it would be possible for my children to be born with a much more severe type and die before the age of two if that happened. Again, I heard her ask, "How are you? What is going through your head right now?"

I could barely form the words, "I'm okay. I guess I'm disappointed that this isn't something that will get better." Disappointed was an understatement. I was devastated. All I wanted to do was get off the phone so I could cry and maybe scream a little too.

This was the last thing I expected. I just wanted to know what I needed to do to be able to fix my muscle problem. I never imagined that the answer would be something they don't have an answer for. Or something that would continue to get worse over time. Something that would mean ending up paralyzed. I didn't even know how to process the information. All this time and I thought I should be happy to have an answer after all these years, but instead I was crushed and confused.

*   *   *

S, M, and A. The three letters that changed my life forever. Before this whole thing started those were simply random letters strung together in an alphabet. No longer a ghost I was trying to hide, I now have a name for my demon. SMA, Spinal Muscular Atrophy, Type 3. A diagnosis. Finally, after all these years. It wasn't in my head, I wasn't crazy. I am not crazy. It was, it is all real. Now, I have to face the facts. Up until this moment, I have survived. Everything I'd ever been through trying to hide a disease and doing a pretty good job at hiding it, I might add. Now, I have a choice to make. Do I keep going, or do I let go?

Nothing the doctors were telling me was making sense. Everywhere I went it was the same thing; a pitied look full of fear for what my life was; what my life is. The only thing I took away, everyone was surprised I can still walk. Why wouldn't I be able to walk? Back to the internet. This time instead of searching "weak and muscles" to try an obtain a diagnosis, I have a name I can search. The lack of results is astonishing.

The only information I am able to find is mostly for SMA Type 1. They told me that I am a Type 3. No wonder everyone I have come in contact with from the medical profession had a panicked look of worry and fear all over their faces. I can't even count the amount of times after the fact that licensed medical doctors have asked me what SMA is when they see it written in my chart. The physical therapists that gave up on me because despite doing the exercises they gave me to do, I wasn't getting any stronger. Right then and there, I made a promise to myself that I would keep on fighting, no matter how hard, no matter what it took, to keep going. I made a promise to myself that I would be able to continue to walk for as long as possible, even if only into my thirties like predicted, and to never, ever, ever give up!

Epilogue

I hung up the phone, jumping for joy and shout, "Yes!" as soon as I jump in my car, so the sound is muffled. Only a couple people at work know what is going on and I'm fairly new to this place, so I'm not ready to reveal the rest of myself. I am identified as completely normal, not the girl with a disability because they still don't know.

Back to the phone, it had been buzzing for the last half hour as the news was coming through. A few people that knew I was anxiously waiting for the news contacted me to let me know. First, I received the text message from Julie, my access manager from the pharmaceutical company. Then, I listened to the voicemail from the physician assistant at the neuromuscular clinic at Stanford. Both delivering the same news, I will be starting Spinraza in less than a month. The only treatment for Spinal Muscular Atrophy had been FDA approved at the very end of the previous year and finally, I had my chance.

All I know is that the medicine is supposed to stop any progression of the disease and I have a chance! I'm glad that I didn't give up those four years ago when they told me I wouldn't have a chance at life. Here I am, still walking like they said I wouldn't be and even still able to jump. Yes, my muscles have weakened a little bit since my diagnosis, but not like they said they would.

I'm also here still working, another thing they said I wouldn't be able to do. If only they could see me now. Maybe I could tell them how to treat patients with dignity and not try and stampede on hope. I am now going to be changing my destiny with a new medication, or at least the destiny that had been set for me.

My life dream has always been to be able to get up from the ground without using my arms to push myself up. Just as I was starting to adjust to the idea that someday I may lose the ability to walk, a miracle comes along. I don't know what is in store for my future, but I do know that at least I can try to gain strength again and all hope will not be lost.

About the Author

At the time of releasing this book, Courtney is 28 years old. She has a bachelor's degree in Business Finance from Southern New Hampshire University and dreams of one day being self-employed. She is still living with Spinal Muscular Atrophy Type 3 and is still able to walk. To date, Courtney has received eight doses of Spinraza. She has seen significant improvements while being on this medication. She writes about her experience with SMA on her blog, www.smainvisiblelife.com. She also shares her experience through her YouTube channel, www.youtube.com/CourtneyFrazer. She has been able to seek support through Cure SMA and has connected with others living with the same disease.

www.ingramcontent.com/pod-product-compliance
Lightning Source LLC
Chambersburg PA
CBHW031151250726

48655CB00002B/933